GASTROINTESTINAL REFLUX DISEASE

(GERD)

How to Manage GERD Disease and Diet So That You Can Live Life to Its Fullest

By **Gavin Sky**

Copyright © 2015 by Gavin Sky

Disclaimers

The information in this book is not intended as medical advice or a substitute for consultation with your healthcare provider. This information should be used in conjunction with the advice of your own healthcare practitioner. Always consult with your physician prior to changing and/or discontinuing medications or diet.

Any trademarks or product names used in this publication are the property of their owners, and are for identification only, and no claim implied by their use.

Table of Contents

Introduction

GERD stands for Gastrointestinal Reflux Disease which is more commonly known as acid or gastric reflux. It is most prevalent among individuals in their thirties and forties and is characterized by what we refer to as heartburn. Anxiety and stress is usually a trigger factor that's why it is most common among the working population age level. But there are other causes apart from these that can lead to GERD and it should be emphasized that GERD is not just a condition. GERD is a disease that should be treated and not ignored or left unattended.

Gastrointestinal reflux disease is very common, affecting up to 1 in 5 or more of adult men and women in the U.S. population. It also occurs in children. Although common, the disease often is unrecognized and its symptoms misunderstood. This is unfortunate because GERD is generally a treatable disease, though serious complications can result if it is not treated properly.

GERD can be triggered by some factors such as food and beverage intake which causes the lower muscles of the esophagus to relax. This results to a heartburn which typically occurs half an hour after taking a heavy meal. A feeling of discomfort begins behind the breastbone and gradually moves up to the area around the throat and neck. This can last for more than 10 minutes and even up to a few hours and may be accompanied by a sour taste that rises from the stomach, some belching and difficulty in swallowing. More advanced effects of GERD include hoarseness, a chronic cough and even asthma.

You should see a specialist if you suspect you have GERD. Although prevention is key to the elimination of the disease, a specialist can provide medication to treat your symptoms and advice you on what you should avoid in order to achieve full recovery. Individuals with GERD are usually advised to stay away from spicy and high-fat diets, citrus and tomatoes and all products containing these, coffee and caffeinated drinks, chocolates, smoking and alcohol among others. It is also advised that people with GERD don't take late night meals or get to bed immediately after eating.

Acid reflux occurs because of the weakening of the muscles in the lower esophagus brought about by certain foods such as diet and behavioral factors. This condition is one of the most common gastrointestinal disorder experienced by a lot of people. It is manifested by several symptoms such as:

Heartburn - this is the burning sensation or dull aching pain felt behind the sternum (breastbone) and radiates even up to the throat and neck area. The pain can be moderate to severe that oftentimes, it is mistaken for a heart attack. This is the most common symptom experienced by about 75% of acid reflux sufferers. It is usually felt at night time after engaging in such activities as bending over, eating heavy meal, lifting heavy objects, doing vigorous exercise or lying down right after eating.

Dyspepsia is another symptom characterized by the feeling of fullness in the upper abdomen sometimes accompanied by recurrent pain, feeling of dizziness and throwing up.

Regurgitation is sensation of acid backing up and producing a sour taste in the mouth. Other symptoms of acid reflux are hoarseness, sore throat, difficulty swallowing, belching, asthma and coughing.

Acid reflux can be treated with dietary changes and lifestyle modifications. You should learn to control the urge for foods that cause you discomfort. Exclude coffee, soda, chocolates, spicy foods, fried foods and foods that have high content as they are bad diet for acid reflux sufferers. If you are a smoker, you should stop it immediately as it can definitely make your situation worse; the same thing with alcohol intake. If you are overweight, you should also start losing weight now as extra fats can cause pressure on the stomach which can lead to the reflux of acid. Proper eating habits should also be observed which includes eating smaller portion of meals instead of big ones and eating at least three hours before bed time.

Though over the counter medications can bring instant relief to you, you should also be aware that it can have side effects in the long run. If you want to be totally free of acid reflux disease, you should take a holistic approach in treating the problem. This includes healing all aspects of your body which are the body, mind, spirit and emotional well-being.

Heartburn is the most frequent but not the only the symptom of GERD. (The disease may be present even without apparent symptoms.) Heartburn is not specific to GERD and can result from other disorders that occur inside and outside the esophagus. All too often, GERD is either self-treated or mistreated.

GERD is a chronic disease. Treatment usually must be maintained on a long-term basis, even after symptoms have been brought under control. Issues of daily living and compliance with long-term use of medication need to be addressed as well. This can be accomplished through follow-up and education.

GERD is often characterized by painful symptoms that can undermine an individual's quality of life. Various methods to effectively treat GERD range from lifestyle measures to the use of medication or surgical procedures.

It is essential for individuals who suffer the chronic and recurrent symptoms of GERD to seek an accurate diagnosis, to work with their physician, and to receive the most effective treatment available.

What is Gastrointestinal Reflux Disease?

Gastrointestinal reflux disease, commonly referred to as GERD or acid reflux, is a condition in which the liquid content of the stomach regurgitates (backs up or refluxes) into the esophagus. The liquid can inflame and damage the lining (cause esophagitis) of the esophagus although visible signs of inflammation occur in a minority of patients. The regurgitated liquid usually contains acid and pepsin that are produced by the stomach. (Pepsin is an enzyme that begins the digestion of proteins in the stomach.) The refluxed liquid also may contain bile that has backed-up into the stomach from the duodenum. (The duodenum is the first part of the small intestine that attaches to the stomach.) Acid is believed to be the most injurious component of the refluxed liquid. Pepsin and bile also may injure the esophagus, but their role in the production of esophageal inflammation and damage is not as clear as the role of acid.

GERD is a chronic condition. Once it begins, it usually is life-long. If there is injury to the lining of the esophagus (esophagitis), this also is a chronic condition. Moreover, after the esophagus has healed with treatment and treatment is stopped, the injury will return in most patients within a few months. Once treatment for GERD is begun, therefore, it usually will need to be continued indefinitely although it is argued that in some patients with intermittent symptoms and no esophagitis, treatment can be intermittent and done only during symptomatic periods.

In fact, the reflux of the stomach's liquid contents into the esophagus occurs in most normal individuals. One study found that reflux occurs as frequently in normal individuals as in patients with GERD. In patients with GERD, however, the refluxed liquid contains acid more often, and the acid remains in the esophagus longer. It has also been found that liquid refluxes to a higher level in the esophagus in patients with GERD than normal individuals.

As is often the case, the body has ways (mechanisms) to protect itself from the harmful effects of reflux and acid. For example, most reflux occurs during the day when individuals are upright.

In the upright position, the refluxed liquid is more likely to flow back down into the stomach due to the effect of gravity. In addition, while individuals are awake, they repeatedly swallow, whether or not there is reflux. Each swallow carries any refluxed liquid back into the stomach. Finally, the salivary glands in the mouth produce saliva, which contains bicarbonate. With each swallow, bicarbonate-containing saliva travels down the esophagus. The bicarbonate neutralizes the small amount of acid that remains in the esophagus after gravity and swallowing have removed most of the acidic liquid.

Gravity, swallowing, and saliva are important protective mechanisms for the esophagus, but they are effective only when individuals are in the upright position. At night during sleep, gravity has no in effect, swallowing stops, and the secretion of saliva is reduced. Therefore, reflux that occurs at night is more likely to result in acid remaining in the esophagus longer and causing greater damage to the esophagus.

Certain conditions make a person susceptible to GERD. For example, GERD can be a serious problem during pregnancy. The elevated hormone levels of pregnancy probably cause reflux by lowering the pressure in the lower esophageal sphincter (see below). At the same time, the growing fetus increases the pressure in the abdomen. Both of these effects would be expected to increase reflux. Also, patients with diseases that weaken the esophageal muscles (see below), such as scleroderma or mixed connective tissue diseases, are more prone to develop GERD.

What Causes Gastrointestinal Reflux Disease?

There is no known single cause of gastrointestinal reflux disease (GERD). It occurs when the esophageal defenses are overwhelmed by gastric contents that reflux into the esophagus. This can cause injury to tissue. GERD can also be present without esophageal damage (approximately 50 – 70% of patients have this form of the disease).

Gastrointestinal reflux occurs when the LES barrier is somehow compromised. Occasional reflux occurs normally, and without consequence other than infrequent heartburn, in people who do not have GERD. In people with GERD, reflux causes frequent symptoms or damages the esophageal tissue.

Some, but not all, people with hiatal hernia have GERD and vice versa. Hiatal hernia occurs when a part of the stomach moves above the diaphragm, from the abdominal to the chest area. The diaphragm is a muscle that separates the chest (containing the esophagus) from the abdomen (containing the stomach). If the diaphragm is not intact, it can compromise the ability of the LES to prevent acid reflux. A hiatal hernia may decrease the sphincter pressure necessary to maintain the anti-reflux barrier.

Even when the LES and the diaphragm are intact and functioning normally, reflux can still occur. The LES may relax after having large meals leading to distension of the upper part of the stomach. When that happens there is not enough pressure at the LES to prevent reflux. In some patients the LES is too weak or cannot mount enough pressure to prevent reflux during periods of increased pressure within the abdomen.

The extent of injury to the esophagus and the degree of severity of GERD depends on the frequency of reflux, the amount of time the refluxed material stays in the esophagus, and the quantity of acid in the esophagus.

What Are The Symptoms Of Uncomplicated GERD?

The symptoms of uncomplicated GERD are primarily heartburn (sometimes interpreted as chest pain), regurgitation, and nausea. Other symptoms occur when there are complications of GERD and will be discussed with the complications.

Heartburn

When acid refluxes back into the esophagus in patients with GERD, nerve fibers in the esophagus are stimulated. This nerve stimulation results most commonly in heartburn, the pain that is characteristic of GERD. Heartburn usually is described as a burning pain in the middle of the chest. It may start high in the abdomen or may extend up into the neck. In some patients, however, the pain may be sharp or pressure-like, rather than burning. Such pain can mimic heart pain (angina). In other patients, the pain may extend to the back.

Since acid reflux is more common after meals, heartburn is more common after meals. Heartburn is also more common when individuals lie down because without the effects of gravity, reflux occurs more easily, and acid is returned to the stomach more slowly. Many patients with GERD are awakened from sleep by heartburn.

Episodes of heartburn may occur infrequently or frequently, but episodes tend to happen periodically. This means that the episodes are more frequent or severe for a period of several weeks or months, and then they become less frequent or severe or even absent for several weeks or months. This periodicity of symptoms provides the rationale for intermittent treatment in patients with GERD who do not have esophagitis. Nevertheless, heartburn is a life-long problem, and it almost always returns.

Regurgitation

Regurgitation is the appearance of refluxed liquid in the mouth. In most patients with GERD, usually only small quantities of liquid reach the esophagus, and the liquid remains in the lower esophagus. Occasionally in some patients with GERD, larger quantities of liquid, sometimes containing food, are refluxed and reach the upper esophagus.

At the upper end of the esophagus is the upper esophageal sphincter (UES). The UES is a circular ring of muscle that is very similar in its actions to the LES. That is, the UES prevents esophageal contents from backing up into the throat. When small amounts of refluxed liquid and/or foods breach (get through) the UES and enter the throat, there may be an acid taste in the mouth. If larger quantities breach the UES, patients may suddenly find their mouths filled with the liquid or food. What's more, frequent or prolonged regurgitation can lead to acid-induced erosions of the teeth.

Nausea

Nausea is uncommon in GERD. In some patients, however, it may be frequent or severe and may result in vomiting. In fact, in patients with unexplained nausea and/or vomiting, GERD is one of the first conditions to be considered. It is not clear why some patients with GERD develop mainly heartburn and others develop mainly nausea.

What Are The Complications Of Gerd?

Ulcers

The liquid from the stomach that refluxes into the esophagus damages the cells lining the esophagus. The body responds in the way that it usually responds to damage, which is with inflammation (esophagitis). The purpose of inflammation is to neutralize the damaging agent and begin the process of healing. If the damage goes deeply into the esophagus, an ulcer forms. An ulcer is simply a break in the lining of the esophagus that occurs in an area of inflammation. Ulcers and the additional inflammation they provoke may erode into the esophageal blood vessels and give rise to bleeding into the esophagus.

Occasionally, the bleeding is severe and may require:

- Blood transfusions,
- An endoscopic procedure (in which a tube is inserted through the mouth into the esophagus to visualize the site of bleeding and to stop the bleeding), or
- Surgical treatment.

Strictures

Ulcers of the esophagus heal with the formation of scars (fibrosis). Over time, the scar tissue shrinks and narrows the lumen (inner cavity) of the esophagus. This scarred narrowing is called a stricture. Swallowed food may get stuck in the esophagus once the narrowing becomes severe enough (usually when it restricts the esophageal lumen to a diameter of one centimeter). This situation may necessitate endoscopic removal of the stuck food. Then, to prevent food from sticking, the narrowing must be stretched (widened). Moreover, to prevent a recurrence of the stricture, reflux also must be prevented.

Barrett's Esophagus

Long-standing and/or severe GERD causes changes in the cells that line the esophagus in some patients. These cells are pre-cancerous and may, though usually, become cancerous. This condition is referred to as Barrett's esophagus and occurs in approximately 10% of patients with GERD. The type of esophageal cancer associated with Barrett's esophagus (adenocarcinoma) is increasing in frequency. It is not clear why some patients with GERD develop Barrett's esophagus, but most do not.

Barrett's esophagus can be recognized visually at the time of an endoscopy and confirmed by microscopic examination of the lining cells. Then, patients with Barrett's esophagus can undergo periodic surveillance endoscopies with biopsies although there is not agreement as to which patients require surveillance. The purpose of surveillance is to detect progression from pre-cancer to more cancerous changes so that cancer-preventing treatment can be started. It also is believed that patients with Barrett's esophagus should receive maximum treatment for GERD to prevent further damage to the esophagus. Procedures are being studied that remove the abnormal lining cells. Several endoscopic, non-surgical techniques can be used to remove the cells. These techniques are attractive because they do not require surgery; however, there are associated with complications, and the long-term effectiveness of the treatments has not yet been determined. Surgical removal of the esophagus is always an option.

Cough and Asthma

Many nerves are in the lower esophagus. Some of these nerves are stimulated by the refluxed acid, and this stimulation results in pain (usually heartburn). Other nerves that are stimulated do not produce pain. Instead, they stimulate yet other nerves that provoke coughing. In this way, refluxed liquid can cause coughing without ever reaching the throat! In a similar manner, reflux into the lower esophagus can stimulate esophageal nerves that connect to and can stimulate nerves going to the lungs. These nerves to the lungs then can cause the smaller breathing tubes to narrow, resulting in an attack of asthma.

Although GERD may cause cough, it is not a common cause of unexplained coughing. Although GERD also may be a cause of asthma, it is more likely that it precipitates asthmatic attacks in patients who already have asthma. Although chronic cough and asthma are common ailments, it is not clear just how often they are aggravated or caused by GERD.

Inflammation of the Throat and Larynx

If refluxed liquid gets past the upper esophageal sphincter, it can enter the throat (pharynx) and even the voice box (larynx). The resulting inflammation can lead to a sore throat and hoarseness. As with coughing and asthma, it is not clear just how commonly GERD is responsible for otherwise unexplained inflammation of the throat and larynx.

Inflammation and Infection of the Lungs

Refluxed liquid that passes from the throat (pharynx) and into the larynx can enter the lungs (aspiration). The reflux of liquid into the lungs (called aspiration) often results in coughing and choking. Aspiration, however, also can occur without producing these symptoms. With or without these symptoms, aspiration may lead to infection of the lungs and result in pneumonia. This type of pneumonia is a serious problem requiring immediate treatment. When aspiration is unaccompanied by symptoms, it can result in a slow, progressive scarring of the lungs (pulmonary fibrosis) that can be seen on chest X-rays. Aspiration is more likely to occur at night because that is when the processes (mechanisms) that protect against reflux are not active and the coughing reflex that protects the lungs also is not active.

Fluid in the Sinuses and Middle Ears

The throat communicates with the nasal passages. In small children, two patches of lymph tissue, called the adenoids, are located where the upper part of the throat joins the nasal passages. The passages from the sinuses and the tubes from the middle ears (Eustachian tubes) open into the rear of the nasal passages near the adenoids. Refluxed liquid that enters the upper throat can inflame the adenoids and cause them to swell. The swollen adenoids then can block the passages from the sinuses and the Eustachian tubes. When the sinuses and middle ears are closed off from the nasal passages by the swelling of the adenoids, fluid accumulates within them. This accumulation of fluid can lead to discomfort in the sinuses and ears. Since the adenoids are prominent in young children, and not in adults, this fluid accumulation in the ears and sinuses is seen in children and not adults.

How is Acid Reflux Diagnosed?

If you experience classic symptoms of acid reflux disease -- chronic heartburn and regurgitation without any troublesome complications, it may be relatively easy for your doctor to make an acid reflux diagnosis.

A few people have GERD that doesn't respond to treatment. Or they may have other concerning symptoms, such as weight loss, difficulty swallowing, anemia, or black stools. If you're one of them, you may need any of the following tests.

Diagnosing Acid Reflux with a Barium Swallow Radiograph

Your doctor may decide to use a special X-ray procedure -- the barium swallow radiograph to rule out any structural problems in your esophagus. In this painless acid reflux test, you will be asked to swallow a solution of barium. The barium enables doctors to take X-rays of your esophagus.

Barium swallow isn't a surefire method of diagnosing GERD. Only one out of every three people with GERD has esophageal changes that are visible on X-rays.

Diagnosing Acid Reflux with Endoscopy or EGD

During an endoscopy, the doctor inserts a small tube with a camera on the end through the mouth into the esophagus. This enables the doctor to see the lining of the esophagus and stomach.

Before inserting the tube, your gastroenterologist may administer a mild sedative to help you relax. The doctor may also spray your throat with an analgesic spray to make the procedure more comfortable for you.

This acid reflux test typically lasts about 20 minutes. It is not painful and will not interfere with your ability to breathe.

While this test may detect some complications of GERD, including esophagitis and Barrett's esophagus, only about half the people with acid reflux disease have visible changes to the lining of their esophagus.

Diagnosing Acid Reflux with a Biopsy

Depending on what the EGD shows, your doctor may decide to perform a biopsy during the procedure. If this is the case, your gastroenterologist will pass a tiny surgical instrument through the scope to remove a small piece of the lining in the esophagus. The tissue sample will then be sent to a pathology lab for analysis. There it will be assessed to see if there is an underlying disease such as esophageal cancer.

Diagnosing Acid Reflux with Esophageal Manometry

Your doctor may perform an esophageal manometry to diagnose acid reflux. This is a test to assess your esophageal function. It also checks to see if the esophageal sphincter, a valve between the stomach and esophagus is working as well as it should.

After applying a numbing agent to the inside of your nose, the doctor will ask you to remain seated. Then a narrow, flexible tube will be passed through your nose, through your esophagus, and into your stomach.

When the tube is in the correct position, the doctor will have you lay on your left side. When you do, sensors on the tube will measure the pressure being exerted at various locations inside your esophagus and stomach. To assess your esophageal functioning even further, you may be asked to take a few sips of water. The sensors on the tube will record the muscle contractions in your esophagus as the water passes down into your stomach. The test typically takes 20 to 30 minutes.

Diagnosing Acid Reflux with Esophageal Impedance Monitoring

To obtain an even more detailed picture of how your esophagus functions, the gastroenterologist may recommend esophageal impedance monitoring. If so, this will be done in conjunction with manometry.

This test uses a manometry tube with electrodes placed at various points along its length. It measures the rate at which liquids and gases pass through your esophagus. When these results are compared with your manometry findings, your doctor will be able to assess how effectively your esophageal contractions are moving substances through your esophagus into your stomach.

Diagnosing Acid Reflux with pH Monitoring

This test uses a pH monitor to record the acidity in your esophagus over a 24-hour period. In one version of this test, a small tube with a pH sensor on the end is passed through your nose into your lower esophagus. The tube is left in place for 24 hours with the portion exiting your nose affixed to the side of your face. It will be connected to a small recording device that you can wear or carry.

During the course of this acid reflux test, you will record in a diary when you are eating or drinking. You will also push a specific button on the recording device to indicate when you are experiencing acid reflux symptoms. This detailed information will allow the doctor to analyze and interpret your test results.

A newer, wireless version of this test is now being used. In this version a small pH sensor is affixed to your lower esophagus using suction. The small probe is able to communicate wirelessly with a recording device outside your body for 48 hours. The probe ultimately falls off and passes through the remainder of the digestive tract.

Many patients have found the wireless pH monitoring exam to be far more pleasant than the traditional version. Both techniques yield similarly information.

How Is GERD Treated?

One of the simplest treatments for GERD is referred to as life-style changes, a combination of several changes in habit, particularly related to eating.

Lifestyle Changes and GERD Diet

As discussed above, reflux of acid is more injurious at night than during the day. At night, when individuals are lying down, it is easier for reflux to occur. The reason that it is easier is because gravity is not opposing the reflux, as it does in the upright position during the day. In addition, the lack of an effect of gravity allows the refluxed liquid to travel further up the esophagus and remain in the esophagus longer. These problems can be overcome partially by elevating the upper body in bed. The elevation is accomplished either by putting blocks under the bed's feet at the head of the bed or, more conveniently, by sleeping with the upper body on a foam rubber wedge. These maneuvers raise the esophagus above the stomach and partially restore the effects of gravity. It is important that the upper body and not just the head be elevated. Elevating only the head does not raise the esophagus and fails to restore the effects of gravity. Elevation of the upper body at night generally is recommended for all patients with GERD. Nevertheless, most patients with GERD have reflux only during the day and elevation at night is of little benefit for them. It is not possible to know for certain which patients will benefit from elevation at night unless acid testing clearly demonstrates night reflux. However, patients who have heartburn, regurgitation, or other symptoms of GERD at night are probably experiencing reflux at night and definitely should elevate their upper body when sleeping. Reflux also occurs less frequently when patients lie on their left rather than their right sides.

GERD Diet

Several changes in eating habits can be beneficial in treating GERD. Reflux is worse following meals. This probably is so because the stomach is distended with food at that time and transient relaxations of the lower esophageal sphincter are more frequent. Therefore, smaller and earlier evening meals may reduce the amount of reflux for two reasons. First, the smaller meal results in lesser distention of the stomach. Second, by bedtime, a smaller and earlier meal is more likely to have emptied from the stomach than is a larger one. As a result, reflux is less likely to occur when patients with GERD lie down to sleep.

Certain foods are known to reduce the pressure in the lower esophageal sphincter and thereby promote reflux. These foods should be avoided and include:

Chocolate

Peppermint

Alcohol, and

Caffeinated drinks.

Fatty foods (which should be decreased) and smoking (which should be stopped) also reduce the pressure in the sphincter and promote reflux.

In addition, patients with GERD may find that other foods aggravate their symptoms. Examples are spicy or acid-containing foods, like citrus juices, carbonated beverages, and tomato juice. These foods should also be avoided if they provoke symptoms.

One novel approach to the treatment of GERD is chewing gum. Chewing gum stimulates the production of more bicarbonate-containing saliva and increases the rate of swallowing. After the saliva is swallowed, it neutralizes acid in the esophagus. In effect, chewing gum exaggerates one of the normal processes that neutralize acid in the esophagus. It is not clear, however, how effective chewing gum is in treating heartburn. Nevertheless, chewing gum after meals is certainly worth a try.

These tips will help with the lessening of your acid reflux disease and its accompanying burning feeling are:

1) You have to change your eating habits. No longer can you indulge in those acidic, fatty foods you may have enjoyed in the past. These foods take much longer to digest and forces

the stomach to produce more acid to aid in this longer digestion period. You also must not stuff yourself with big meals but have more, smaller meals. Also do not eat anything three or four hours before going to bed. While you are standing gravity helps prevent the stomach acid from going up into the esophagus. When lying flat in bed the lower esophageal sprinter has a better chance of opening and allowing this acid and undigested food to enter the esophagus

2) You must avoid tight-fitting clothes. Don't wear any slimming devices and tight-fitting belts that will apply pressure to the stomach and force it to push undigested food and acid up into the esophagus. If you feel you are overweight then diet and mild exercise are much better for you than trying to force your stomach to appear slimmer by using these tight-fitting devices.

3) Avoid stress as much as possible as it adds to the development of acid in your stomach. If you feel stressed, the best thing you can do for it is to relax and go for a brisk walk. This will not only help reduce your stress but is great for your overall health by lowering your weight and cholesterol level and increasing your heart rate. So, you get several benefits from this one activity.

So even if acid reflux is a life-long condition, you can, with a few adjustments in your living habits lower or even wipe out the dreadful effects of this disease. The changes you have to make are much easier to cope with than the burning feeling you will suffer with GERD. Follow these tips and make the necessary changes today.

GERD Friendly Recipes

GERD does not need to be tasteless and dull when it comes to meal time. With some planning ahead, GERD is manageable at meal time. Below are listed some of the foods that should be avoided when managing your diet with GERD:

Chocolate

Onions

Fried Foods

Fatty Foods

Garlic

Chili Peppers

Coffee

Caffeinated Beverages

Tomato and Citrus Juices

Instead of having the ingredients listed above, try adding foods that have more fiber in your diet.

Eating smaller meals frequently instead of large meals is definitely a benefit that will help manage increased acid production.

Muesli Style Oatmeal

Ingredients

1 cup instant oatmeal

1 cup milk

2 tbsp. raisins (brought to a boil, drained)

½ banana, diced

½ golden apple, peeled, diced

Pinch of salt

2 tsp. sugar or honey

Directions

1. The evening before (or at least 2 hours before), mix the oatmeal, milk, raisins, salt, and sugar (or honey) together in a bowl.

2. Cover and place in the refrigerator.

3. Add fruit before serving.

4. If the mix is too thick, add milk.

Ginger Banana Smoothie

Ingredients

½ cup ice

2 cups milk

2 bananas, ripe

1 cup yogurt

½ tsp. fresh ginger, peeled and grated fine

2 tbsp. brown sugar or honey (optional)

Directions

1. In a blender, add the ice, milk, yogurt, bananas, and ginger.

2. Blend until smooth.

3. Add sugar as needed.

Crispy Baked Buttermilk Chicken Strips

When avoiding fried food such as Chicken Strips, try is oven baked recipe instead:

Ingredients:

1 pound chicken tenders

1 cup low-fat buttermilk

1 tablespoon canola oil (for greasing bottom of baking sheet)

3/4 cup unbleached flour

1/2 teaspoon fresh cracked black pepper (if tolerated)

1/2 teaspoon salt

1/4 cayenne pepper (if tolerated)

1 cup panko breadcrumbs

Canola cooking spray

Directions:

1.   Wash the chicken tenders and dry well with paper towels. Place chicken pieces and buttermilk in medium-sized covered bowl and refrigerate for at least 30 minutes or overnight.
2.   Preheat oven to 400-degrees. Spread the canola oil over the bottom of a 9 x 13-inch baking dish.
3.   Place flour, pepper, salt, and cayenne pepper in a shallow bowl and whisk to blend ingredients. Place Panko crumbs in a shallow bowl and line up the bowls and pan in this order: flour mixture then chicken then Panko crumbs then prepared baking dish.
4.   Place one piece of chicken in the seasoned flour, then dip the chicken back into the buttermilk briefly. Place chicken in Panko crumbs next, and then place in prepared baking dish. Repeat with remaining chicken tenders. Coat top of chicken strips generously with canola cooking spray.

5.   Bake in center of oven for about 25 minutes or until chicken is nicely browned on the outside and cooked throughout on the inside. Remove from oven and serve with desired sauces or condiments that are well tolerated.

In general, people with a tendency to have heartburn might react to condiments/sauces containing tomato based products, chili pepper, Tabasco, mustard seed, curry powder, and fresh garlic.

Yield: Makes about 8 chicken strips

Per strip:124 calories, 14.5 g protein, 7.5 g carbohydrate, 3.5 g fat, .7 g saturated fat, 1.7 g monounsaturated fat, 1 g polyunsaturated fat, 36 mg cholesterol, .2 g fiber, 116 mg sodium. Calories from fat: 25 percent. Omega-3 fatty acids = .2 gram, Omega-6 fatty acids = .6 gram

Artichoke Heart, Spinach Dip

Ingredients:

Alfredo Sauce:

1 tablespoon extra-virgin olive oil

2 cups low-fat milk, divided (whole milk or fat-free half and half can also be used)

4 tablespoons unbleached white flour or Wondra quick-mixing flour

1/8 teaspoon ground nutmeg (if tolerated)

1/8 teaspoon white pepper (if tolerated)

1/3 cup shredded Parmesan cheese

1 tablespoon minced or chopped garlic (if tolerated)

1/4 cup chopped green onions (if tolerated)

10-ounce package frozen chopped spinach, thawed and gently squeezed of excess water

2 cups chopped artichoke hearts, water packed or thawed from frozen, drained and chopped (marinated artichoke hearts can be used if drained well)

1 cup shredded part-skim mozzarella cheese

Directions:

1. Preheat oven to 350-degrees. Coat an 8 x 8-inch baking dish with canola cooking spray.

2. Make Alfredo sauce by whisking together olive oil, 1/3 cup of the milk, 4 tablespoons flour, nutmeg and pepper to medium, nonstick saucepan. Slowly stir in remaining milk. Bring mixture to a gentle boil over medium-high heat then reduce heat to medium-low and continue to gently boil, stirring constantly until sauce thickens (about 2 minutes). Stir in 1/3-cup shredded Parmesan cheese.

3. Add garlic, green onions, spinach, artichoke hearts, Alfredo sauce, and mozzarella cheese to a large mixing bowl and stir to blend with a spoon.

3. Spread mixture into an 8 x 8-inch baking dish and bake until bubbly (about 30 minutes). Serve warm with bite-size pieces of whole wheat sourdough bread or whole grain crackers or tortilla chips.

Yield: Makes 12 servings

Per serving (just the dip): 98 calories, 7 g protein, 9 g carbohydrate, 4 g fat, 2 g saturated fat, 1.5 g monounsaturated fat, .3 g polyunsaturated fat, 9 mg cholesterol, 3 g fiber, 130 mg sodium. Calories from fat: 37 percent.

Omega-3 fatty acids = .1 g Omega-6 fatty acids = .2 g

Hummus

Ingredients

1 can (19 oz.) canned chickpeas (drained and washed twice)

1 cup chicken stock

2 tbsp. olive oil

¼ tsp. sesame oil

½ tsp. salt

Directions

1. Place the chickpeas in a food processor and add the chicken stock, olive oil,sesame oil, and salt.

2. Process until smooth.

3. Add chicken stock as needed.

4. Serve cold with toast points, oven-toasted corn chips, or small wedges of flatbread.

Macaroni Salad

This is a high-fiber meal that has a lightly seasoned dressing and low-fat. Feel free to add ingredients that will only compliment this wonderful recipe.

Ingredients:

3 hard-boiled eggs, higher omega-3 if possible

2 cups dry whole wheat macaroni noodles

2 teaspoons parsley flakes or 2 tablespoons fresh, finely chopped parsley

1/4 teaspoon salt

Freshly ground pepper to taste and as tolerated

3 tablespoons real or light mayonnaise

1/3 cup nonfat plain Greek yogurt (fat free sour cream can be substituted)

Optional Additions: (if tolerated):
3 finely chopped green onions (white and part of green)
1/4 cup finely chopped celery
1/4 cup finely chopped sweet or dill pickles

Directions:

1. Boil Eggs. Boil macaroni noodles, following directions on box (noodles usually need 8 minutes to boil). Drain noodles well, rinse, and let cool.
2. Place noodles in serving bowl along with parsley, salt and pepper to taste, and any optional additions that are well tolerated.
3. In small bowl, blend mayonnaise with Greek yogurt well, then stir into the noodle mixture in serving bowl.
4. Peel shells off eggs and remove half of the yolks. Chop remaining eggs and stir into the macaroni mixture. Cover and let macaroni salad sit in refrigerator overnight (if time permits).

Yields: 8 side servings

Per serving: 129 calories, 6 g protein, 22 g carbohydrate, 2.4 g fat, .5 g saturated fat, .9 g monounsaturated fat, 1 g polyunsaturated fat, 41 mg cholesterol, 2.2 g fiber, 142 mg sodium. Calories from fat: 17 percent. Omega-3 fatty acids = .1 gram Omega-6 fatty acids = .8 gram

Slow Cooker Chicken Dinner

Ingredients

4 TBSP packed brown sugar
4 TBSP white wine
4 TBSP red wine vinegar (divided)
2 TBSP dried oregano
3 bay leaves
1 teaspoon celery salt
1/2 tsp pepper
2 TBSP capers with a bit of juice
1/2 cup large pitted Spanish green olives cut in half
1 cup prunes
8 small chicken legs bone in (about 4 pounds split with skin removed)
1/4 cup chopped fresh parsley or chopped cilantro

Directions

1. In a large slow cooker whisk together the brown sugar, oregano, wine, 2 TBSP of vinegar with 1/2 cup of water, and add salt and pepper.

2. Add bay leaves, capers, olives, and prunes, and stir well.

3. Place the chicken pieces in the pot and surround them with the olives and prunes.

4. Cover and cook on low for 5 to 6 hours or on high for 3 to 4 hours.

5. Thirty minutes before serving, gently mix in parsley or cilantro and remaining 2 TBSP vinegar.

6. Remove chicken when ready and place on a platter with prunes and olives.

7. Reserve liquid, heat, and pour into a sauce boat to serve over rice.

Nutritional information (per serving): Calories 220, Sat fat 2 g, Sodium 385 mg

Makes 6-8 Servings

Trout Almondine

Ingredients

1-1/4 TBSP olive oil
1/2 teaspoon dried basil
1/2 teaspoon ground ginger
4 trout fillets
2 large red, yellow or green bell peppers
1/3 cup sliced unsalted almonds
4 lemon wedges (omit if it triggers your GERD symptoms)

Directions

1. Preheat the broiler to high.

2. Whisk oil and herbs together in a small bowl. Line a broiler pan with foil and brush lightly with the oil.

3. Arrange the fish fillets skin side down on foil in the center of the pan.

4. Slice the peppers into 1/2 inch slices and place them around the fish.

5. Brush the trout and peppers with prepared oil and broil for 2 to 3 minutes. Turn the fillets over and brush with more oil. Continue to broil for another 2 to 3 minutes until bubbling or beginning to crisp.

6. Carefully place almonds on top of the fish and broil for a minute or less until golden brown.

7. Transfer to plates and serve immediately.

Nutritional information (per serving): Calories 365, Sat fat 3g, Sodium 35 mg

Serves 4

Chicken and Dumplings

Ingredients

For the stew:
1 pound skinless, boneless chicken meat, cut into 1-inch cubes
1/2 cup onion, coarsely chopped*
1 medium carrot, peeled and thinly sliced
1 stalk celery, thinly sliced
1/4 tsp salt
Black pepper to taste
1 pinch ground cloves
1 bay leaf
3 C water
1 tsp cornstarch
1 tsp dried basil
1 package (10 oz) frozen peas

For the cornmeal dumplings:
1 C yellow cornmeal
3/4 C sifted all-purpose flour
2 tsp baking powder
1/2 tsp salt
1 C low-fat (1%) milk
1 Tbsp vegetable oil

Directions

Directions for the stew:

1. Place chicken, onion*, carrot, celery, salt, pepper, cloves, bay leaf, and water in a large saucepan.

2. Heat to boiling; cover and reduce heat to simmer. Cook about 1/2 hour or until chicken is tender.

3. Remove chicken and vegetables from broth. Strain broth.

4. Skim fat from broth; measure and, if necessary, add water to make 3 cups liquid.

5. Mix cornstarch with 1 cup cooled broth by shaking vigorously in a jar with a tight-fitting lid.

6. Pour into saucepan with remaining broth; cook, stirring constantly, until mixture comes to a boil and is thickened.

7. Add basil, peas, and reserved vegetables to sauce; stir to combine.

8. Add chicken and heat slowly to boiling while preparing cornmeal dumplings.

Directions for the dumplings:

1. Sift together cornmeal, flour, baking powder, and salt into a large mixing bowl.

2. Mix together milk and oil.

3. Add milk mixture all at once to dry ingredients; stir just enough to moisten flour and evenly distribute liquid. Dough will be soft.

4. Drop by full tablespoons on top of braised meat or stew.

5. Cover tightly; heat to boiling. Reduce heat (do not lift cover) to simmering and steam about 20 minutes.

*Omit onion if cooked onion triggers your GERD symptoms, or replace it with an appropriate amount of the dried form.

Nutritional information (per serving): Calories 307, Total fat 5 g, Saturated fat 1 g, Cholesterol 43 mg, Sodium 471 mg

Baked French Fries

Makes 5 servings--Serving size: 1 cup

Ingredients

4 large Russets or Idaho potatoes (2 lbs)
8 cups ice water
Apple cider vinegar
1 tsp garlic powder*
1 tsp onion powder*
1/4 tsp salt
1 tsp white pepper
1/4 tsp allspice
1 Tbsp vegetable oil

Directions

1. Scrub potatoes and cut into long 1/2-inch strips.

2. Place potato strips into ice water, cover, and chill for 1 hour or longer.

3. Remove potatoes and dry strips thoroughly.

4. Place garlic powder, onion powder, salt, white pepper, allspice, and pepper flakes in a plastic bag.

5. Toss potatoes in spice mixture.

6. Brush potatoes with oil.

7. Place potatoes in nonstick shallow baking pan.

8. Cover with aluminum foil and place in 475° F oven for 15 minutes.

9. Remove foil and continue baking uncovered for an additional 15 to 20 minutes or until golden brown and crispy!

10. Turn fries occasionally to brown on all sides.

Nutritional information (per serving): Calories 238, Fat 4 g, Saturated fat 1 g, Cholesterol 0 mg, Sodium 163 mg

Beef and Mushrooms

Yield: 5 servings--Serving Size: 6 oz

Ingredients

1 pound lean beef (top round)
3 TBSP apple cider vinegar
2 tsp vegetable oil
3/4 TBSP dried minced onion* (do not use if triggers GERD symptoms)
1 pound sliced mushrooms
1/4 tsp salt
pepper to taste
1/4 tsp nutmeg
1/4 tsp ginger
1/2 tsp dried basil
1/4 C white wine
1 C plain low-fat yogurt
6 C cooked macaroni, cooked in unsalted water

Directions

1. Cut beef into 1-inch cubes, and marinate for at least 2 hours in vinegar.

2. Heat 1 teaspoon oil in a non-stick skillet.

3. Add beef and sauté for 5 minutes. Turn to brown evenly. Remove from pan and keep hot.

4. Add remaining oil to pan; sauté mushrooms.

5. Add beef to pan with seasonings.

6. Add wine, yogurt, and dried onion; gently stir in. Heat, but do not boil.

7. Serve with whole wheat pasta or brown rice

Note: If thickening is desired, use 2 teaspoons cornstarch; calories are the same as flour, but it has double thickening power. These calories are not figured into the nutrients per serving.

Nutritional Information (per serving): Calories: 499, Total fat: 10 g, Saturated fat: 3 g Cholesterol: 79 mg, Sodium: 200 mg

6772129R00025

Printed in Germany
by Amazon Distribution
GmbH, Leipzig